Stay Strong and Confident

Easy Exercises for Enhancing Strength and Confidence for Seniors 2024

By

FRED D. DAVIS

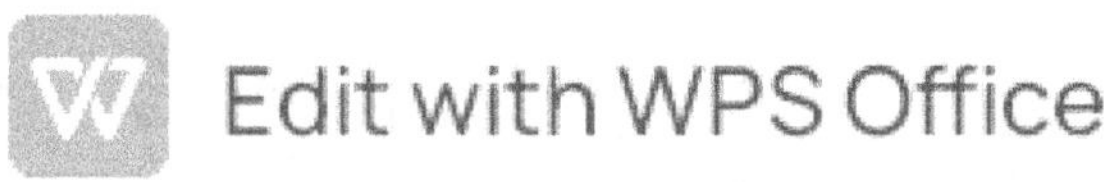

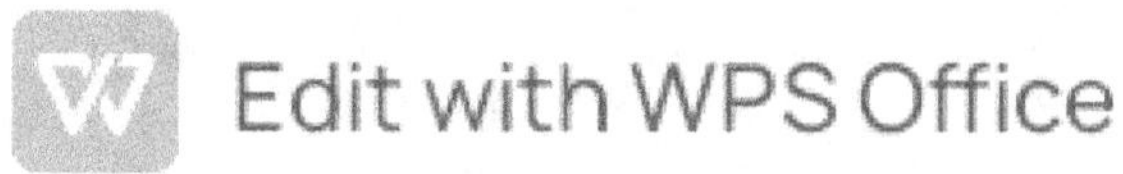
Edit with WPS Office

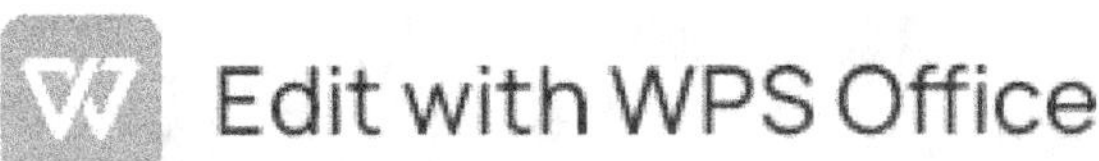

Table of Contents

Fred D. Davis is a seasoned fitness instructor and wellness advocate who is committed to enabling seniors to live vibrant, active lives. With over 20 years of experience in the health and fitness sector, Fred brings a lot of knowledge, passion, and expertise to his work, motivating countless others to prioritise their health and well-being.   7

Fred's fitness journey began with a strong desire to assist others in accomplishing their wellness goals. Recognizing the special requirements and obstacles that seniors confront, he set out on a quest to create accessible, effective exercise programs that are geared specifically to

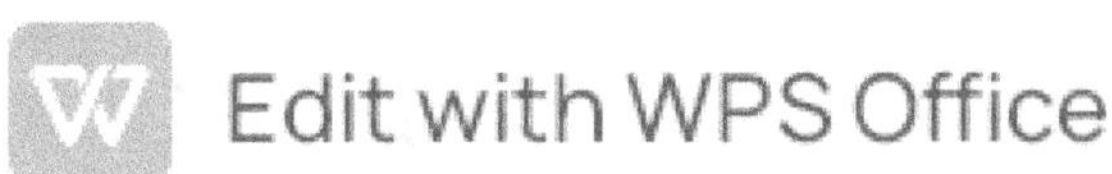

them.8

In his pioneering book, Stay Strong and Confident: Easy Exercises for Enhancing Strength and Confidence for Seniors 2024, Fred shares his wealth of knowledge and skills, providing a thorough approach to improving strength, confidence, and overall well-being in the elderly population. Fred, who has years of experience working with seniors of all fitness levels, introduces a series of simple exercises to develop mobility, muscle strength, and self-confidence.   8

Fred enables elders to take control of their health and embrace the transforming potential of exercise by using a compassionate approach and straightforward, succinct training. With a focus on safety, accessibility, and enjoyment, his book gives seniors the tools and strategies they need to be active, independent, and resilient as they get older.

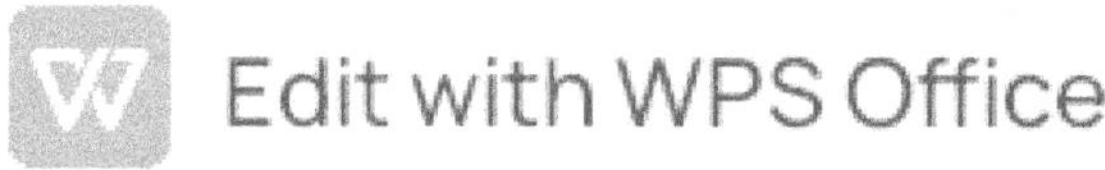

Fred's commitment to promoting senior well-being goes beyond the pages of his book. As a popular speaker and workshop leader, he travels the country, sharing his knowledge and inspiring audiences to adopt healthy habits and live their best lives at any age. 8

Fred Davis' Stay Strong and Confident encourages seniors on a journey of self-discovery, empowerment, and vitality. With his advice and support, readers find that age is no barrier to power, confidence, and limitless vitality. Fred's work continues to have a significant impact on the lives of seniors all around the world, empowering them to remain strong, confident, and resilient as they enjoy the benefits of ageing gracefully.   8

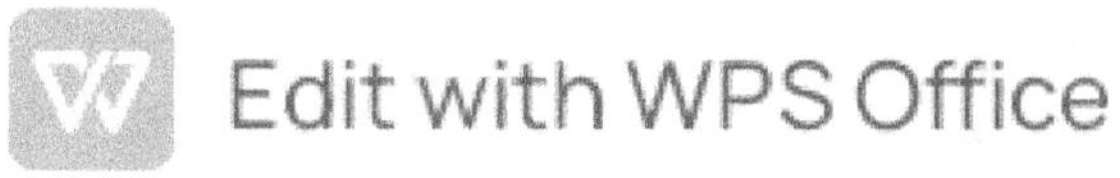

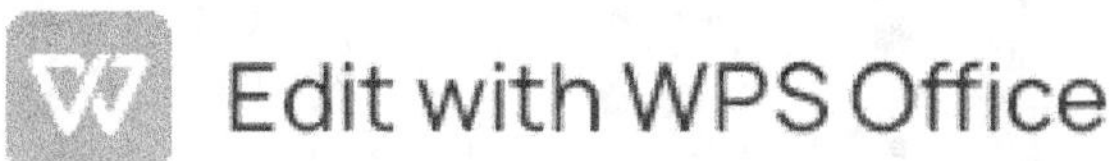

ABOUT THE AUTHOR

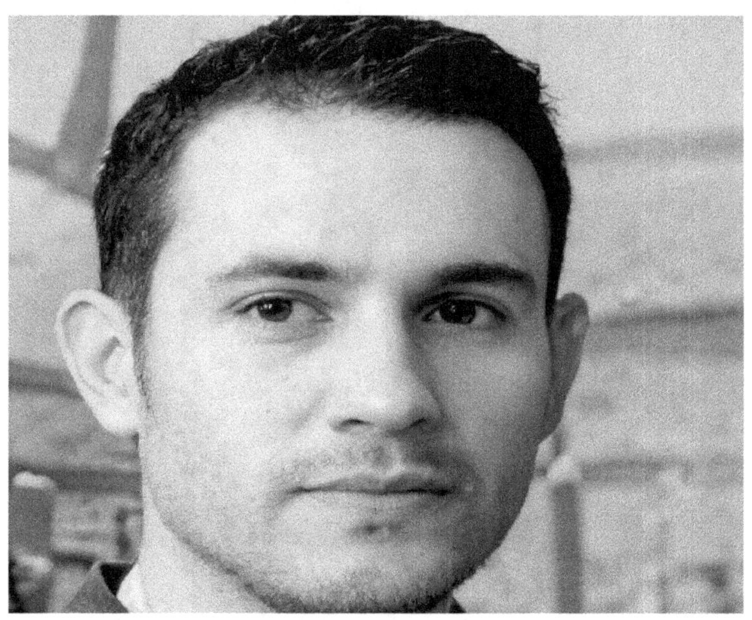

Fred D. Davis is a seasoned fitness instructor and wellness advocate who is committed to enabling seniors to live

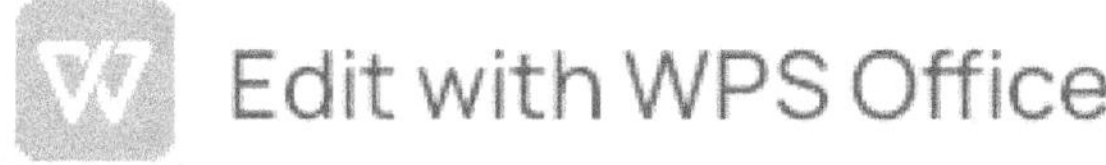

vibrant, active lives. With over 20 years of experience in the health and fitness sector, Fred brings a lot of knowledge, passion, and expertise to his work, motivating countless others to prioritise their health and well-being.

Fred's fitness journey began with a strong desire to assist others in accomplishing their wellness goals. Recognizing the special requirements and obstacles that seniors confront, he set out on a quest to create accessible, effective exercise programs that are geared specifically to them.

In his pioneering book, Stay Strong and Confident: Easy Exercises for Enhancing Strength and Confidence for Seniors 2024, Fred shares his wealth of knowledge and skills, providing a thorough approach to improving strength, confidence, and overall well-being in the elderly population. Fred, who has years of experience working with

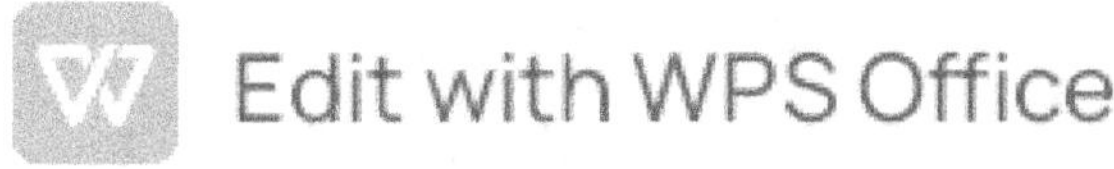

seniors of all fitness levels, introduces a series of simple exercises to develop mobility, muscle strength, and self-confidence.

Fred enables elders to take control of their health and embrace the transforming potential of exercise by using a compassionate approach and straightforward, succinct training. With a focus on safety, accessibility, and enjoyment, his book gives seniors the tools and strategies they need to be active, independent, and resilient as they get older.

Fred's commitment to promoting senior well-being goes beyond the pages of his book. As a popular speaker and workshop leader, he travels the country, sharing his knowledge and inspiring audiences to adopt healthy habits and live their best lives at any age.

Fred Davis' Stay Strong and Confident

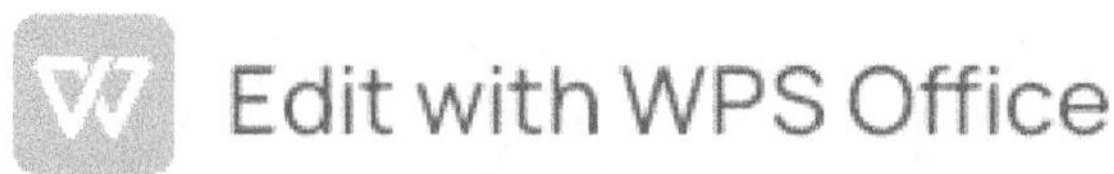

encourages seniors on a journey of self-discovery, empowerment, and vitality. With his advice and support, readers find that age is no barrier to power, confidence, and limitless vitality. Fred's work continues to have a significant impact on the lives of seniors all around the world, empowering them to remain strong, confident, and resilient as they enjoy the benefits of ageing gracefully.

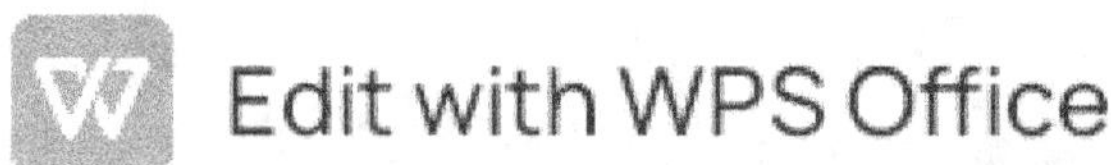

Chapter One
INTRODUCTION

Importance of strength and confidence in elders

As people age, it becomes increasingly important for them to preserve both physical strength and mental clarity. Strength enables seniors to carry out daily activities independently, lowers the chance of injury, and improves general well-being. Simultaneously, confidence is essential for maintaining a positive attitude, conquering obstacles, and accepting new experiences. This book recognises the importance of seniors' strength and confidence and tries to provide helpful insights and information to help them acquire these essential characteristics.

The goal of this book is to provide complete guidance for seniors wishing to improve their strength and confidence via exercise.

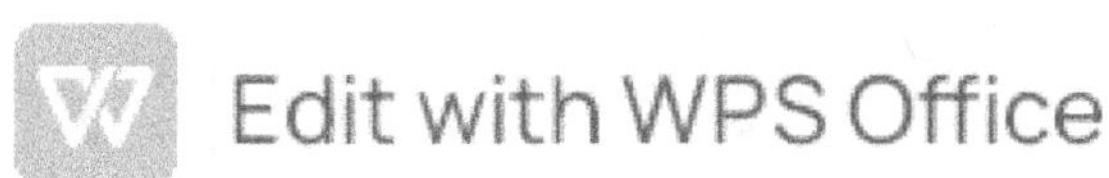

It will provide useful guidance, ideas, and exercises that may be readily integrated into their everyday routines. By can reap a variety of benefits, including improved physical health, more vitality, improved emotional well-being, and a boost in self-confidence.

This book is designed specifically for seniors who are committed to living an active and satisfying life. This book is appropriate for people of all fitness levels and abilities, whether they have been physically active their entire lives or are just beginning out in fitness. It recognises the particular requirements and challenges that elders confront and offers specialised counsel to properly handle these aspects. This book's content is intended to be accessible, instructive, and motivating to seniors with a variety of backgrounds, fitness levels, and aspirations.

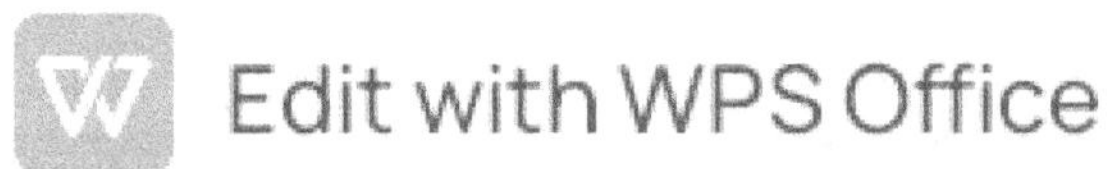

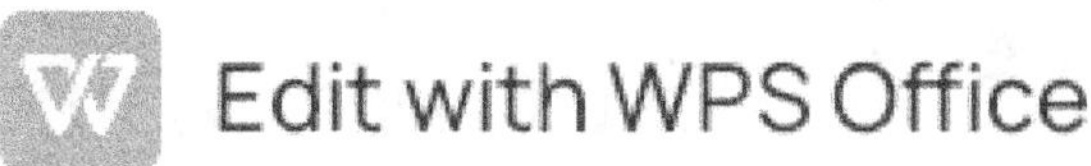

Chapter 2

Understanding Ageing and its Impact on Strength and Confidence.

Exercise can be quite beneficial in reducing the effects of ageing on strength and confidence. Here's a full description of how exercise might be beneficial:

1. Muscle Loss Prevention

As people age, they lose muscle mass. Sarcopenia, or muscle loss, can result in diminished strength, mobility, and general functional ability. Regular exercise, particularly resistance training, promotes muscle growth and maintenance, hence preventing muscle loss. Seniors can improve their physical performance by participating in activities such as weightlifting, resistance band exercises, or bodyweight exercises.

2. Bone Health Improvement

Osteoporosis, a disorder characterised by low bone density and an increased risk of fracture, is also frequently connected with ageing. Exercise, particularly weight training, helps to promote bone health, lower the incidence of fractures, strengthen existing bones, and increase total bone density.

3. Functional independence

Maintaining independence as we age is frequently a major priority. Regular exercise can substantially help you achieve this aim. Functional exercises, which mirror ordinary movements, can help improve balance, flexibility, and coordination. Seniors can enhance their functional fitness with exercises like tai chi, yoga, or Pilates, helping them to accomplish daily tasks more easily and lowering their risk of falling.

4. Cognitive enhancement

Research has demonstrated that exercise improves cognitive performance and mental wellbeing. Regular physical activity boosts blood flow to the brain, encourages neuroplasticity, and improves memory and cognitive ability. Aerobic exercise, such as brisk walking or cycling, has been shown to improve cognitive capacities such as attention, information processing, and problem-solving.

5. Mood and Confidence Boost

Aging can sometimes be accompanied by feelings of solitude, depression, and decrease dancing effects, boosting the release of endorphins, also known as "feel-good" hormones. This can result in enhanced mental health, increased self-esteem, and a stronger sense of self. Regular brisk walks with friends can also provide opportunities for social

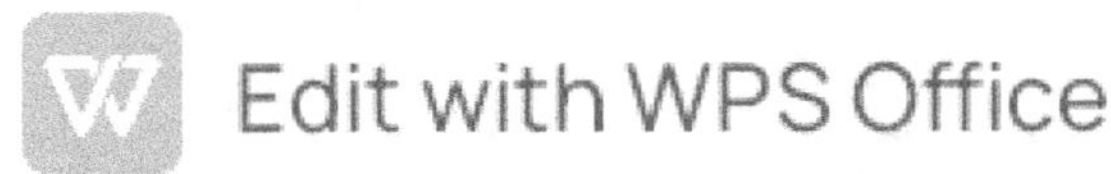

engagement and support while exercising.

6. Decreased muscle mass

As we age, our overall strength and physical ability decline, which has an impact on bone health, with decreased bone density increasing the risk of fractures and osteoporosis. This can have an impact on one's confidence when completing physical activities.

7 . Joint issues

Ageing can cause decreased flexibility and increased joint stiffness, making it more difficult to move and perform specific jobs. This can have an impact on both physical strength and overall confidence.

8 . Changes in balance and coordination

As people age, their balance and coordination skills deteriorate, increasing the danger of falling and injuring themselves. This may result in a loss of

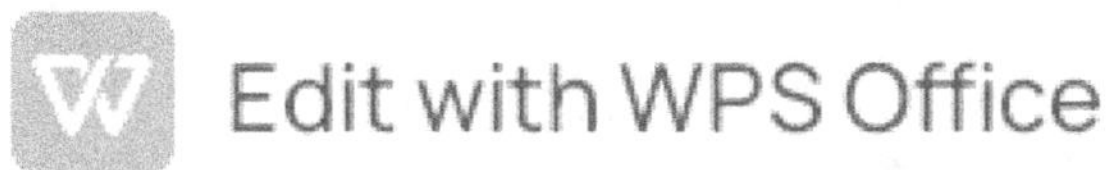

confidence and a fear of participating in physical activities.

9 . Hormonal changes

Hormonal changes associated with ageing, such as decreasing testosterone and oestrogen levels, can cause a reduction in muscle strength and energy. This can have an impact on one's general physical health, often leading to the development of chronic health disorders such as heart disease or diabetes. These diseases can have an impact on strength, mobility, and general confidence when participating in physical activities.

10. Psychological aspects

Ageing might have an impact on confidence because of psychological variables such as vulnerability and societal stereotypes about ageing. These circumstances can lead to a decline in physical strength and confidence.

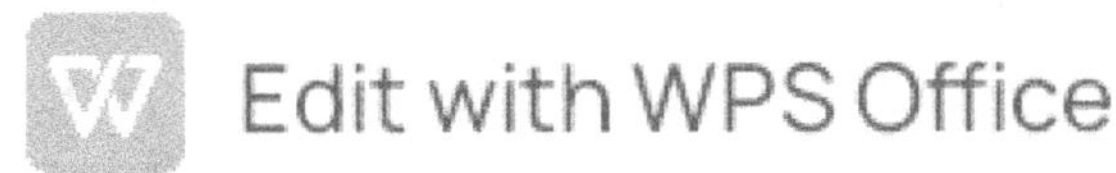

In addition, regular exercise has numerous physical and emotional benefits for elders. It prevents muscle loss, promotes bone health, increases functional independence, and builds confidence. Seniors who incorporate exercise into their daily routine can boost their confidence, leading to a healthier and more happy living.

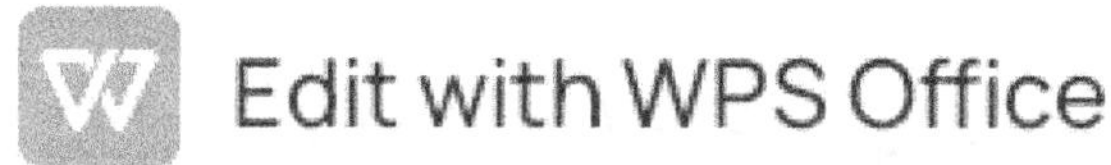

Chapter Three
Benefits of Exercise for seniors

Exercise can have numerous benefits for seniors, both physically and psychologically. Here are some detailed explanations of the benefits:

Physical benefits

. Increased muscle strength and endurance

Regular exercise helps seniors build stronger muscles and improves their overall physical strength. This can make daily tasks easier to perform and reduce the risk of falls or injuries.

. Improved flexibility and balance

Exercise programs that focus on stretching and balance exercises can help seniors improve their flexibility and balance. This can enhance their mobility, reduce the risk of falls, and maintain independence.

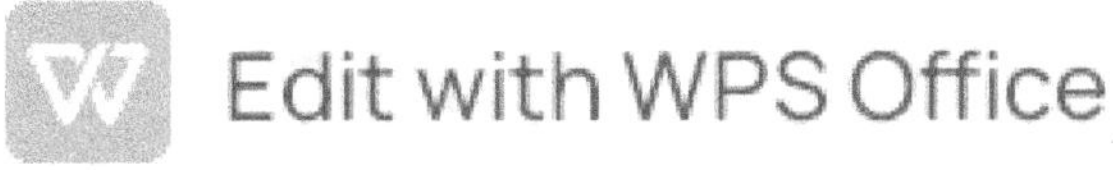

. Enhanced overall fitness levels

Engaging in cardiovascular exercises, such as brisk walking, swimming, or cycling, can improve seniors' cardiovascular health, increase stamina, and contribute to an overall sense of well-being.

Psychological benefits

. Boosted self-esteem and self-confidence

Regular exercise can help seniors feel a sense of accomplishment and boost their self-esteem. As they see improvements in their physical abilities and overall fitness, they often gain confidence in their capabilities.

. Reduced anxiety and depression

Exercise releases endorphins, which are natural mood enhancers. Seniors who exercise regularly often experience a reduction in symptoms of anxiety and depression and may have improved mental

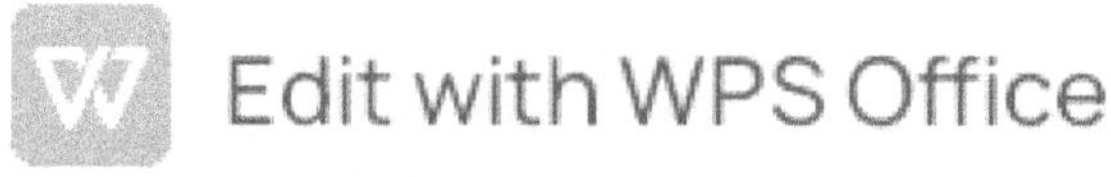

well-being.

. Increased mental sharpness and cognitive function

Research suggests that exercise can benefit brain health, improving memory, attention, and cognitive function. Seniors who engage in physical activity often experience better cognitive performance and a reduced risk of cognitive decline.

Overall, exercise is a crucial component of a healthy lifestyle for seniors. It not only helps them maintain physical fitness but also promotes mental well-being and cognitive function. Senior individuals should consult with healthcare professionals or exercise specialists to develop a personalised exercise plan appropriate for their needs and abilities.

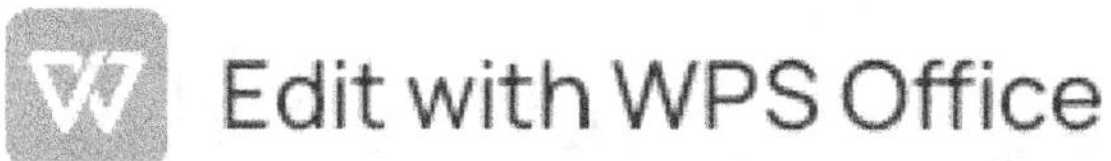

Chapter Four
Designing an Exercise Programme for Seniors

A. Evaluate individual talents and limitations.

•Health Assessment

Seniors should contact a healthcare expert before beginning any exercise programme. This may include a physical examination, a review of your medical history, and measures of flexibility, muscle strength, and overall fitness level.

•Functional Capacity Evaluation

Evaluating the aged person's ability to conduct activities of daily living (ADLs) such as walking, standing up from a chair, or leaning down will assist in determining their baseline functional capability.

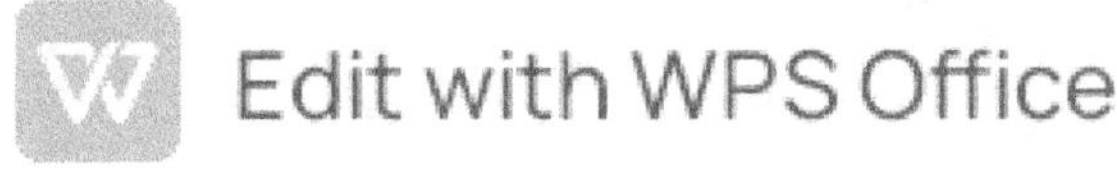

•Balance and Fall Risk Assessment

Assessing balance and recognising fall risks is critical for creating an exercise plan that focuses on strength and stability to prevent falls and injuries.

B. Setting reasonable goals

•Individualised Approach

Set realistic short- and long-term goals based on each senior's goals, preferences, and current fitness level. For some, it may be improving mobility, while others may strive to develop strength or flexibility.

•Gradual Progression

Begin with realistic goals and progressively increase the intensity, duration, and complexity over time. This ensures that ongoing improvement occurs without taxing the individual's talents.

Tailoring activities to meet unique needs

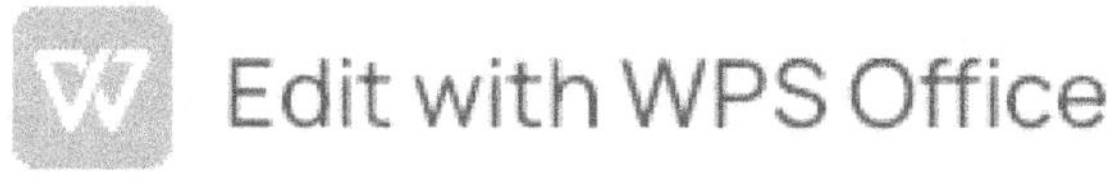

- **Cardiovascular Endurance**

Aerobic workouts like brisk walking, swimming, or cycling can help enhance heart and lung fitness while also supporting overall cardiovascular health.

- **Strength Training**

Include bodyweight, resistance bands, or low weights resistance workouts to maintain or enhance muscle strength. Concentrate on the key muscular groups: legs, arms, chest, back, and core.

- **Flexibility and Range of Motion**

Stretching activities should be used to increase joint flexibility and range of motion. This can involve static stretches, yoga, tai chi, and Pilates.

- **Balance and Coordination**

Include activities that improve balance and coordination skills, such as a toe walk or

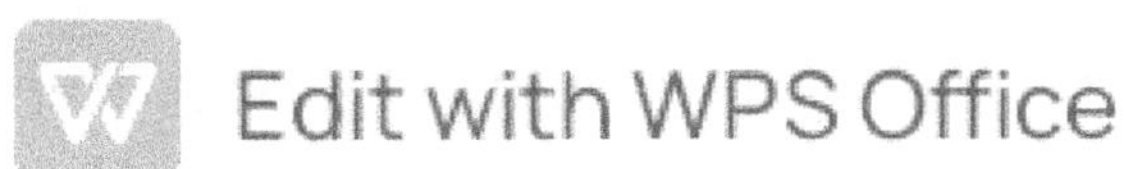

workouts using balance boards or stability balls.

● **Safety precautions and changes**

• Warm up and cool down.

Each stitch in life's exquisite tapestry reflects a moment of care, a regard for the temple of our body. As we approach our elderly years, the discipline of fostering wellness becomes a spiritual practice, a hymn to vitality, resilience, and the timeless grace of ageing gracefully.

The ritual of warm-up and cool-down is crucial to this noble pursuit, an ancient waltz between preparation and meditation, action and quiet, where we honour our bodies' rhythms with gentle care.

For seniors, the warm-up marks the start of a spiritual journey, a gentle invitation to awaken dormant muscles, coax tight joints

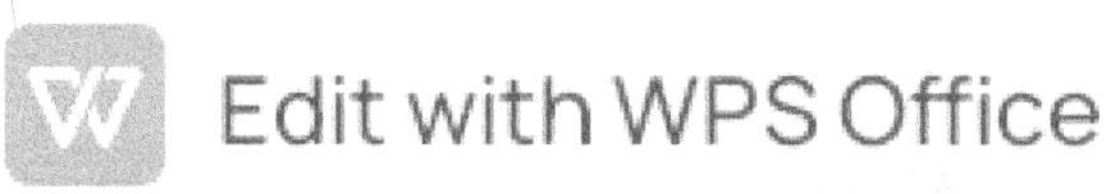

into fluid action, and reignite the spark of vitality that flickers within. It is a time for connection with the body, a silent discourse between flesh and soul that invites us to listen, honour, and embrace the wisdom of our physical form.

The warm-up transforms into a sanctuary, where stress melts away, anxieties fade into the ether, and the sheer joy of movement reigns supreme. It demonstrates the resiliency of the human spirit, our ability to adapt, grow, and thrive in the embrace of mindful motion.

However, as the dance of life progresses, we must also honour its conclusion: the soft rhythm of the cool-down, a graceful retreat into the sanctuary of stillness. The cool-down, like the setting sun shedding its golden glow on the globe, invites us to revel in the afterglow of movement to savour the pleasure of exertion while surrendering to the gentle embrace of repose.

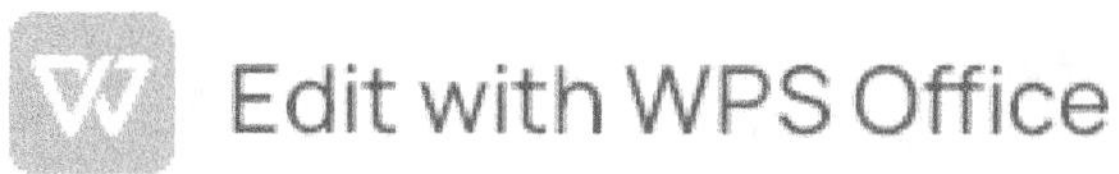

The cool-down transforms into a sanctuary with gentle stretches, relaxing breathwork, and focused reflection, a sanctuary where fatigued muscles find solace, restless minds find quiet, and movement echoes linger like whispers on the breeze. It is a moment of grace, a time when the barriers between body and soul melt, leaving us with nothing but the pure essence of being.

Dear reader, as we embark on the sacred journey of ageing, let us recognize the warm-up and cool-down routines as sacred rites of passage gateways to vitality, resilience, and the timeless beauty of the human spirit. Let us honour our bodies' knowledge, our spirits' resilience, and the limitless potential that every one of us possesses.

•**Use proper form.**

Emphasise the significance of keeping appropriate form during exercises to ensure

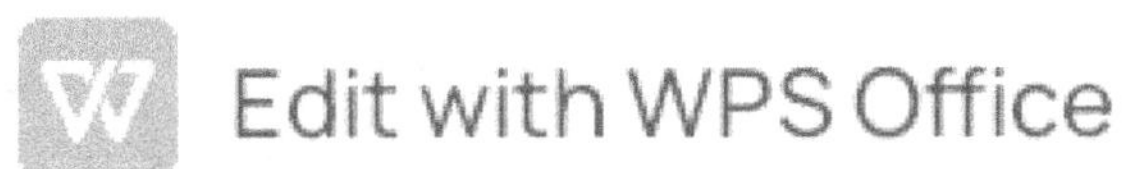

safety and efficacy. This may necessitate guidance from a certified exercise specialist or physical therapist.

Adjust exercise intensity and duration based on an individual's fitness level and any specific constraints. Instead of pushing too hard right away, it is better to gradually increase the difficulty.

• **Monitor vital signs**

Seniors should be conscious of their own bodies and check their heart rate, blood pressure, and overall level of comfort while exercising. If they experience any discomfort or odd indications, they should immediately cease and seek medical attention.

In the journey of life, as we traverse through the golden years, the guardianship of our health becomes ever more crucial. Among the myriad tools at our disposal, the monitoring of vital signs emerges as a

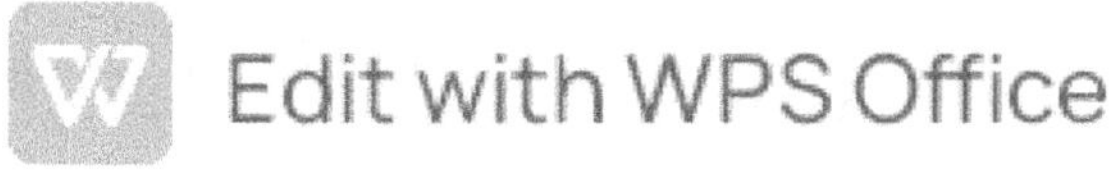

beacon of vigilance, a compass guiding us through the labyrinth of ageing with wisdom and grace.

Vital signs serve as silent sentinels, offering insights into the intricate symphony of our physiological well-being. From the rhythmic cadence of our heartbeat to the ebb and flow of our blood pressure, these subtle indicators paint a portrait of our internal landscape, revealing clues that might otherwise elude our perception.

For seniors, the monitoring of vital signs takes on heightened significance, a lifeline tethering them to a realm of proactive health management and informed decision-making. With advancing age comes a myriad of physiological changes, some subtle, others profound, each bearing its imprint on the delicate tapestry of our vitality.

Consider, for instance, the silent crescendo

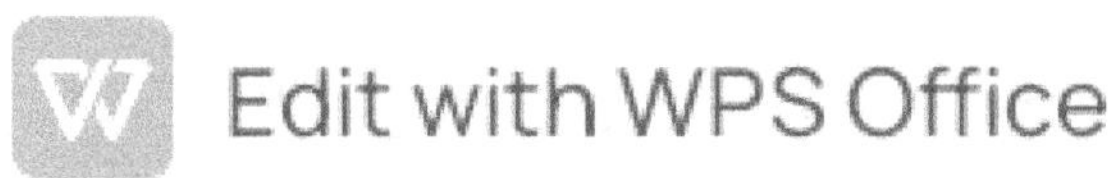

of hypertension a silent assailant stealthily encroaching upon the corridors of our cardiovascular health. Through regular monitoring of blood pressure, seniors can unmask this hidden threat, empowering themselves and their caregivers with the knowledge needed to intervene and mitigate risks.

Similarly, the rhythm of our heartbeat, a symphony conducted by the intricate dance of electrical impulses, holds invaluable insights into the health of our cardiovascular system. Irregularities in heart rate or rhythm may signify underlying conditions warranting further investigation and intervention.

Yet, vital signs extend beyond the realm of cardiovascular health, encompassing a spectrum of physiological parameters that collectively illuminate the landscape of our well-being. From body temperature to respiratory rate, from oxygen saturation to

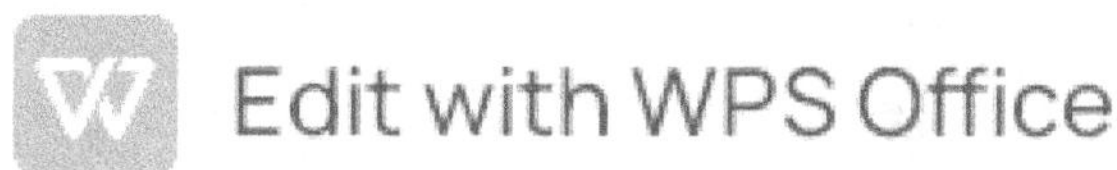

blood glucose levels, each metric offers a unique window into the complex interplay of bodily functions.

But the monitoring of vital signs transcends the realm of mere numbers. it embodies a profound ethos of care and compassion, a commitment to honouring the sanctity of life in all its myriad manifestations. It speaks to a deeper truth that our bodies are not mere vessels but sacred temples deserving of reverence and attention.

Dear reader, as we embark upon the voyage of ageing, let us embrace the mantle of stewardship entrusted to us. Let us pledge ourselves to the noble task of monitoring vital signs not as a burden, but as a sacred duty bestowed upon us by virtue of our humanity.

Let us cultivate a culture of vigilance, where the rhythms of our bodies are revered as sacred hymns echoing the eternal song of

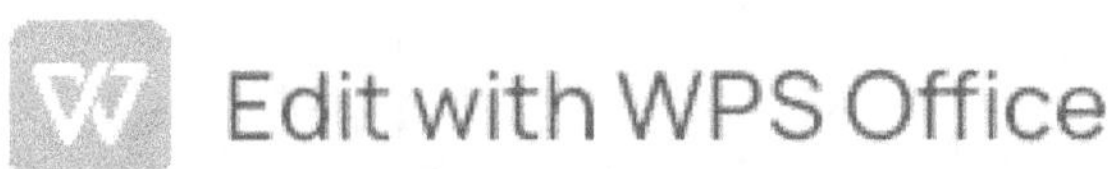

life. Let us stand as guardians of health, steadfast and unwavering in our commitment to the well-being of ourselves and those entrusted to our care.

In the tapestry of existence, the monitoring of vital signs emerges as a luminous thread, a testament to our resilience, our wisdom, and our enduring spirit. May we honour it, cherish it, and let it illuminate the path towards a future imbued with vitality and grace.

•Stay hydrated

Encourage elders to drink water before, during, and after exercise to stay hydrated, particularly in hot or humid weather.

•Avoid overexertion and fatigue

In the maelstrom of modern life, where duties pile up and calendars overflow, it's easy to get caught up in a never-ending loop of activity. However, amidst the

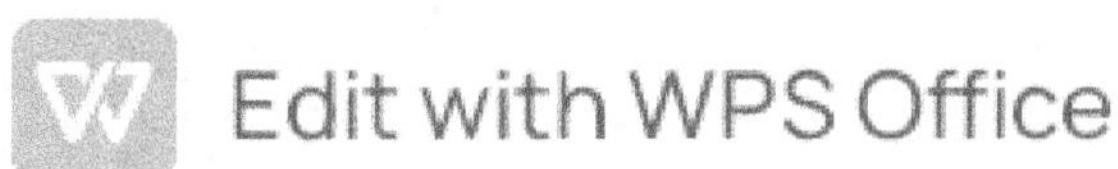

commotion, it is critical to pause and focus on the tremendous importance of protecting our physical and mental health.

Overexertion and weariness are sneaky opponents that lurk in the shadows of our hectic lives, ready to strike when least expected. They manifest not only as physical weary, but also as mental fatigue, depriving us of vigour and delight.

Imagine a life in which every day feels like a war against exhaustion, and even the most basic activities become Herculean challenges. This is the reality for many people who ignore their bodies' and minds' subtle signals, pushing themselves to their limits in order to meet productivity or societal standards.

But it does not have to be this way.

We can liberate ourselves from the bonds of overexertion and exhaustion by practising mindfulness and taking a holistic

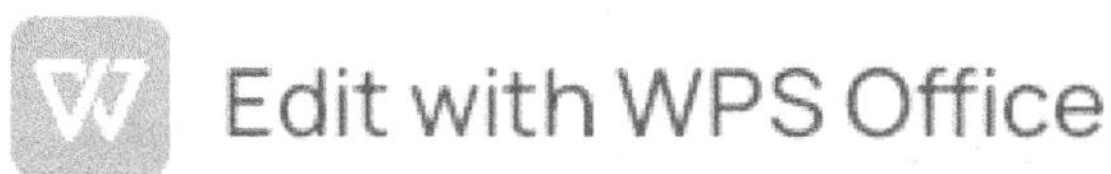

approach to wellness. It starts with appreciating the complex interplay between our physical, emotional, and mental dimensions—a delicate balance that necessitates nurturing and care.

Physical health is the foundation of our well -being. As we age, our bodies change dramatically, prompting changes in our lifestyle and habits. Regular exercise, decent nutrition, and adequate rest are not luxuries, but rather critical pillars of health.

Exercise does not have to be tough or difficult; even simple exercises such as strolling, yoga, or tai chi can energise the body and boost the spirit. Similarly, fueling our bodies with nutritious foods increases our energy stores and strengthens our resistance to weariness.

However, physical health is insufficient until we address the complexities of our mental and emotional landscapes. The mind, like a

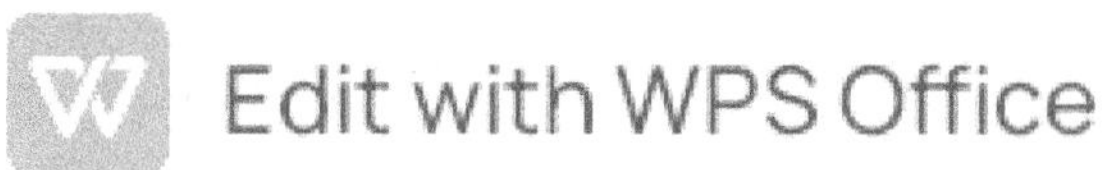

delicate ecosystem, requires care and nourishment to survive. Stress management, relaxing techniques, and developing meaningful relationships with others are all essential components of mental health.

Recognising the symptoms of overexertion and weariness is the first step towards regaining control of our lives. Physical symptoms such as prolonged exhaustion, muscle soreness, or difficulties sleeping should not be ignored, but rather interpreted as urgent requests for attention and self-care.

Equally essential are our psyche's subtle whispers, such as sensations of overwhelm, irritation, or a loss of interest in previously cherished activities. These emotional indicators are helpful guides, pushing us to rethink our priorities and take a kinder, more sympathetic attitude to life.

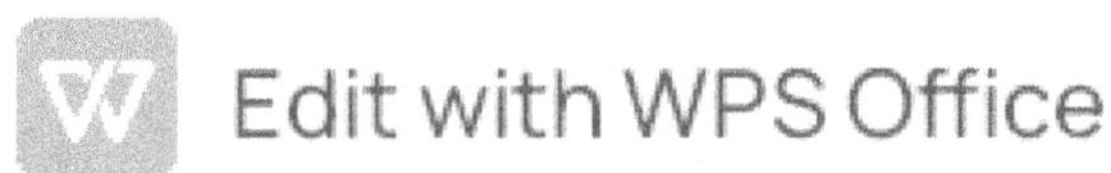

Preventing overexertion and weariness necessitates a holistic approach that includes not just individual self-care routines but also systemic changes in our society standards and expectations. It is a collaborative effort that requires solidarity and support from communities, workplaces, and legislators alike.

Dear reader, as you negotiate the maze of life's problems, I beseech you to listen to your body's wisdom and respect the sacredness of your health. Embrace balance as a guiding principle, incorporating relaxation and rejuvenation into your everyday routine.

Remember that the route to vitality is a marathon, not a sprint—a slow unfolding of self-discovery and growth. Accept the process, enjoy your accomplishments, and be compassionate with yourself during times of failure.

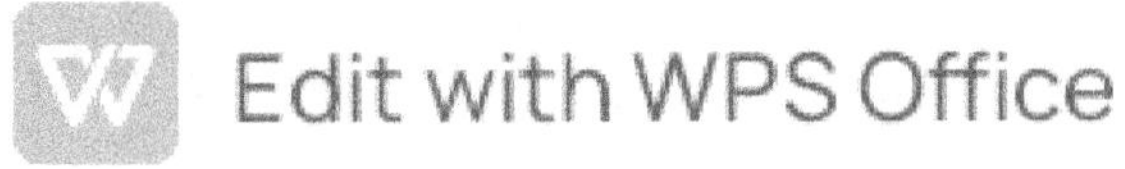

Your well-being is the most valuable thread in the fabric of existence; respect it, cultivate it, and allow it to weave its magic into every part of your life.

Seniors should use caution and avoid overexertion or pushing oneself beyond their limits. Encourage children to pay attention to their bodies and take rest periods as needed.

Remember, elders should speak with healthcare professionals or exercise specialists who can provide personalised advice based on their specific requirements and skills.

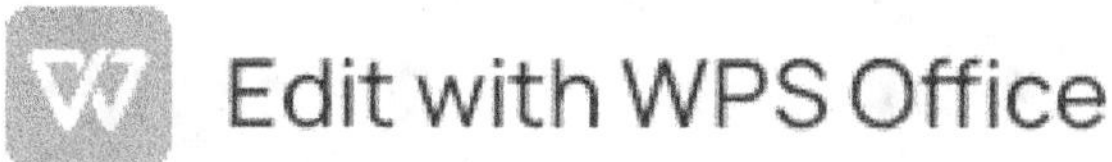

Chapter Five

Easy Exercises to Increase Strength and Confidence

A.Strength exercises.

●Upper Body Workouts

•.Arm Curls.

- Sit or stand holding a lightweight dumbbell in either hand.

- Lift the weights slowly towards your shoulders, using your biceps.

- Lower the weights carefully to finish one repetition.

●Lower Body Exercises.

•Squats

Stand with your feet shoulder-width apart and lower into a sitting position while keeping your back straight.

- Get back up, activating your thighs and

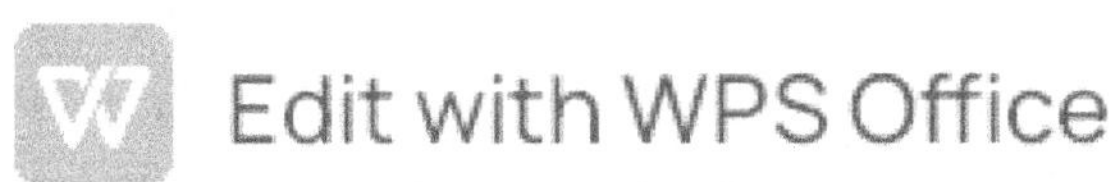

glutes.

- Repeat for a basic yet effective lower-body workout.

• Lunges

•Begin with one foot ahead and lower your hips until your knees are bent at a 90-degree angle.

- Return to the beginning posture, then swap legs to work various muscle groups.

Core Exercises

•Planks

Begin in a push-up position, supporting your body with your forearms.

- Keep your body in a straight line from head to heels while activating your core.

- Maintain the position for as long as you feel comfortable.

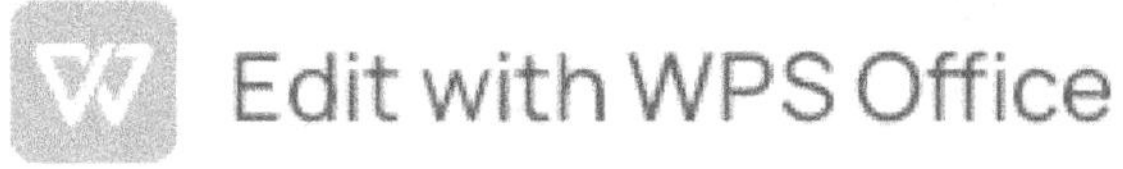

Bridges

-Lie on your back, knees bent, feet flat on the floor.

- Squeeze your glutes as you lift your hips towards the ceiling.

- Lower your hips back to the ground.

B.Balance and Flexibility Exercises

•Yoga poses

•Tree pose

 Stand on one leg and place the sole of the other foot against the inner thigh or calf.

- Place your palms together in front of your chest and hold for balance.

- Switch legs and repeat.

•Warrior pose

 Take one step back while maintaining the front leg bent.

- Stretch your arms out to the sides in a straight line.

 Switch sides to improve balance and leg strength

•Tai Chi Movements

Use slow, flowing movements like &quit;Cloud Hands Quit; and &quit;

Wave Hands Like Clouds Quit; to improve balance and flexibility.

• Stretching routines

Use dynamic stretches to warm up and static stretches to cool down.

- Concentrate on major muscle groups, holding each stretch for 15-30 seconds. Cardiovascular exercises.

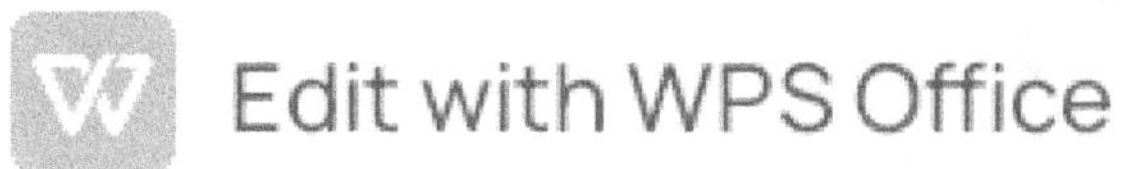

1.Low-impact activities.

Brisk Walking

 - Aim for 30 minutes of brisk walking most days of the week.

- Wear appropriate footwear and maintain a healthy posture.

 - Swimming is a low-impact exercise that works the entire body.

- Vary your strokes to engage different muscle groups.

2. **Stationary Bike or Elliptical Workouts**

•**Stationary Bike**

 - Ride at a moderate pace, adjusting the resistance as necessary . Maintain correct posture to prevent strain.

•Elliptical

- Use both your arms and legs for a low-impact, full-body workout.

- Change the resistance level for a more challenging experience.

3. Water aerobics or Group Fitness Classes

Water Aerobics

Buoyancy decreases joint stress, making it suitable for the elderly .

Classes frequently incorporate aerobics, strength exercises, and stretching.

Attending senior classes develops a friendly environment . Options may include dancing, aerobics, or strength training. These exercises provide a well-rounded approach by developing strength, balance, flexibility, and cardiovascular health in seniors, so improving both physical well-

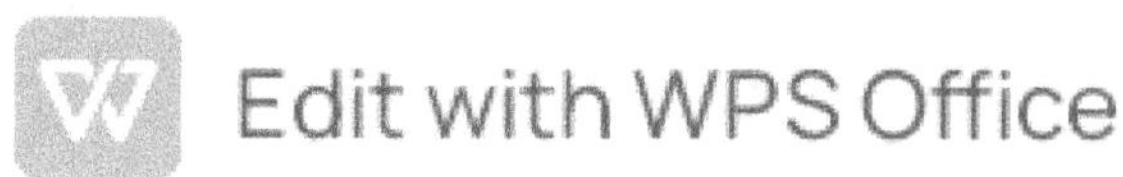

being and confidence. Before beginning any new workout routine, always consult a healthcare expert.

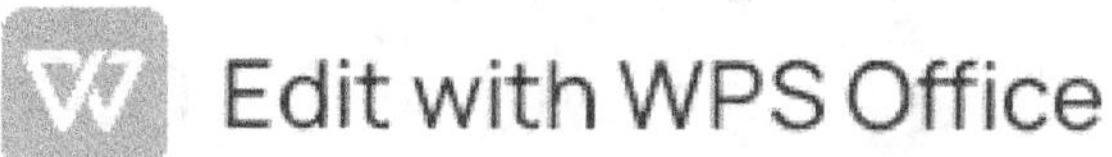

Chapter Six

Incorporating Exercise into Everyday Life

A.Establishing a Regular Exercise Routine

-Set particular times for workouts to establish a consistent regimen.

-Select activities that match your preferences and fitness goals.

- Begin with moderate durations and gradually increase intensity.

B. Sustaining Motivation

- Establish realistic and quantifiable fitness goals to monitor progress.

- Change up the exercises to keep the training interesting and avoid boredom.

- Celebrate accomplishments and milestones to promote a good attitude.

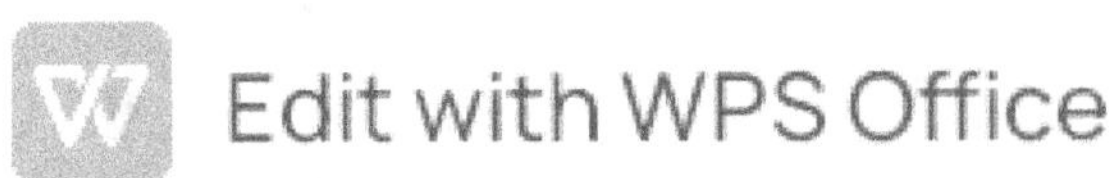

C. Developing Social Support and Accountability

- Exercise with friends or participate in group fitness sessions to boost motivation.

- Share your fitness goals with someone you trust to generate accountability.

- Use exercise apps or online forums to get support and motivation.

Including exercise in daily life is an important part of sustaining general health and well-being, regardless of age. Regular physical activity provides various benefits, including increased strength, better cardiovascular health, improved mood, and a lower chance of chronic diseases.

One method for incorporating exercise into daily life is to prioritise activities that require movement. This can be as simple as using the stairs instead of the lift, walking or biking short distances instead of driving, or performing physical labour-intensive household activities such as gardening or cleaning. These activities not only serve to develop physical strength, but they also add to overall calorie expenditure throughout the day.

Those who like a more planned workout programme should look for a pleasurable and sustainable kind of exercise. This could involve jogging, swimming, dance, yoga, or strength training. To ensure long-term adherence, consider activities that match individual tastes and talents.

 Additionally, bringing exercise into daily life may necessitate making minor changes to daily behaviours. Setting out specific time for physical activity, whether in the morning, during lunch breaks, or in the evening, can help you develop a consistent exercise habit. This could be taking a fitness class, participating in group sports, or simply

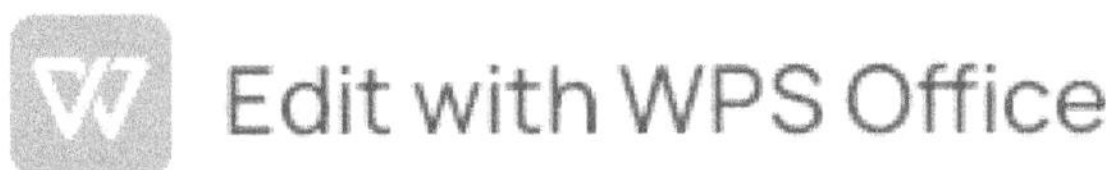

scheduling time for a home workout.

It's also a good idea to ask for the help of family and friends when exercising in your daily routine. Participating in physical activities together not only boosts motivation but also instil a sense of responsibility. This can be accomplished by creating workout buddy systems, joining neighbourhood fitness clubs, or incorporating loved ones in outdoor recreational activities.

Furthermore, technology can be used to aid exercise integration. Fitness applications, smartwatches, and other wearable devices can generate personalised training regimens, track progress, and provide reminders to be active throughout the day. It's a wonderful tool for those who struggle to maintain consistency or require additional motivation.

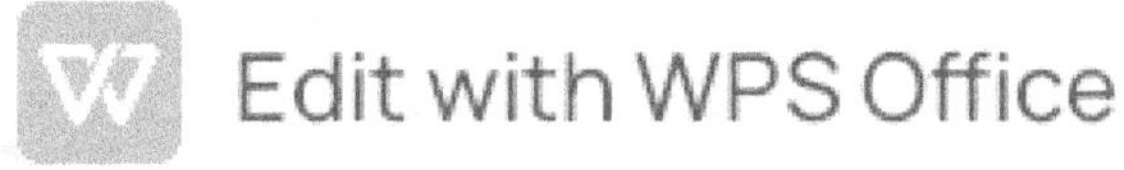

Finally, it is critical to be aware of one's limitations and listen to the body. Starting with low-intensity workouts and gradually increasing the intensity and length will help you avoid injuries and maintain a consistent fitness regimen. Before beginning any new workout programme, it is critical to check with healthcare specialists or fitness experts, particularly if you have pre-existing health ailments or concerns.

Incorporating exercise into daily life is a lifelong commitment to preserving physical strength, boosting general health, and increasing confidence. Individuals can build a sustainable workout regimen by identifying fun activities, making minor changes to daily routines, gathering assistance, utilising technology, and being sensitive to individual limitations.

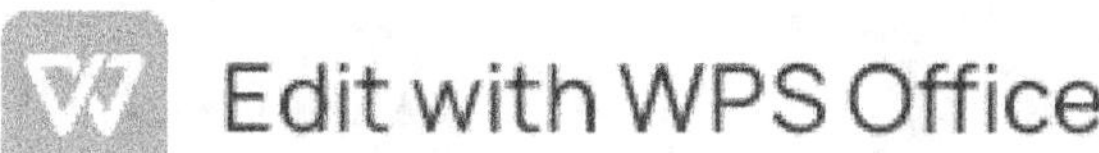

Chapter Seven

Nutrition and Hydration for Maximum Strength and Confidence.

A.The Importance of a Balanced Diet

As you elegantly navigate the lovely path of ageing, allow us to highlight the deep importance of keeping a balanced diet adapted to your specific needs. Your health is a valuable asset, and a well-balanced diet is essential for maintaining vigour, resilience, and overall health

- Choose a variety of fruits, vegetables, whole grains, and lean proteins.

- Include healthy fats, such as avocados and almonds, to improve general health

- Maintain portion management to meet nutritional needs while avoiding excess calories.

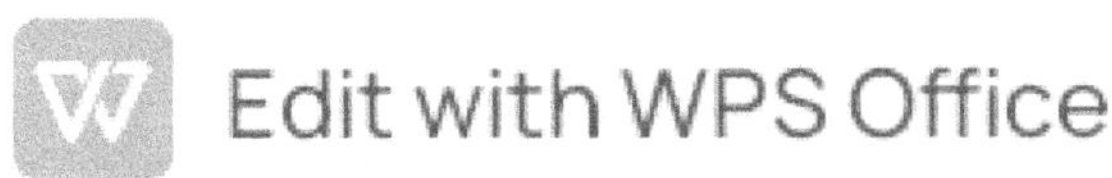

Nutritional Vitality

A healthy diet is your constant companion, delivering the nutrients your body requires to thrive. From vitamins and minerals to protein and fibre, each nutrient boosts your energy, strengthens your immune system, and supports your body's delicate operations, allowing you to face each day with vigour.

Preserving Strength and Mobility

As time passes, it becomes increasingly important to preserve strength and mobility. A well-balanced diet high in lean proteins, calcium, and vitamin D supports your muscles, bones, and joints, keeping strength and flexibility as you enjoy the benefits of exercise and freedom.

Promoting Cognitive Health

Your mind is a beautiful jewel that needs loving care and nutrition. A well-balanced

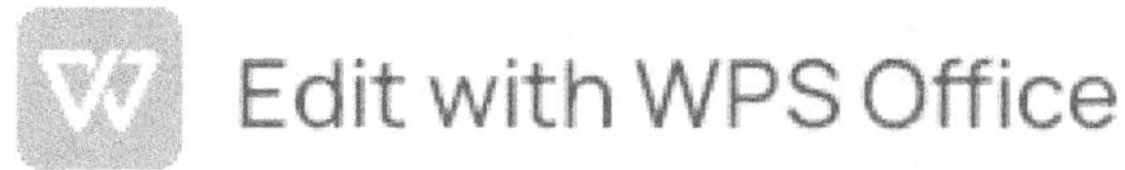

diet rich in antioxidants, omega-3 fatty acids, and brain-boosting nutrients protects your cognitive health by sharpening your memory, improving your focus, and fostering your mental clarity as you embark on new adventures and revisit old ones.

Boosting Heart Health

Your heart is a sturdy protector of life, worthy of loving love and care. A well-balanced diet low in saturated fats and sodium but high in heart-healthy nutrients like fibre, potassium, and unsaturated fats promotes cardiovascular health, lowering your risk of heart disease, stroke, and other cardiovascular conditions while allowing your heart to beat with strength and resilience.

Enhancing Quality of Life

Finally, a balanced diet improves your quality of life by filling each moment with vitality, joy, and well-being. It nourishes your

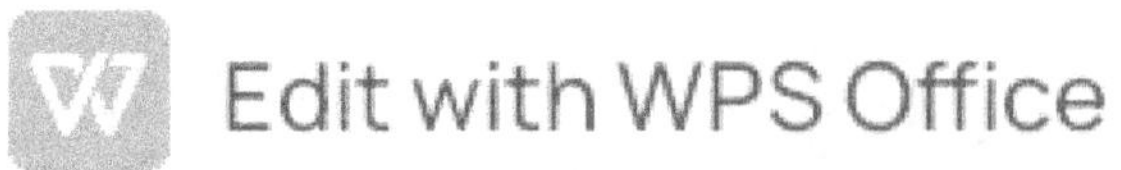

body, soul, and spirit, empowering you to live life to the fullest with grace, gratitude, and unbounded excitement.

B. Recommended Nutrients for Seniors

Calcium & amp; Vitamin D Dairy products and fortified foods contain essential nutrients for bone health.

Fibre

promotes digestive health; resources include whole grains, fruits, and vegetables. Protein Lean meats, fish, legumes, and dairy products are all essential for muscle health. Vitamin B 12 Fish, pork, and fortified grains all include this essential nutrient for neuron function.

Omega 3 Fatty Acids

Fish, flaxseeds, and walnuts all include nutrients that promote heart health.

C. Hydration Guideline

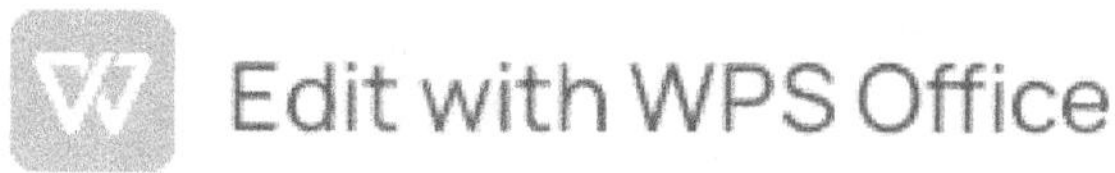

As we age, staying hydrated becomes more vital for our overall health and well-being. Dehydration can cause a wide range of health problems, including urinary tract infections, disorientation, weariness, and even kidney stones. That is why it is critical for seniors to adhere to a hydration schedule to ensure they are consuming adequate fluids throughout the day.

Here are some hydration guidelines that seniors should consider:

1. Aim to consume at least 8-10 cups of fluid per day, which can include water, herbal tea, fruit juice, milk, and broth-based soup. Remember that other liquids, such as coffee and alcohol, might have a diuretic impact, so drink them in moderation.

2. Be aware of your thirst cues

As we age, our sensation of thirst may fade, making it easy to forget to drink adequate water. Make a conscious effort to drink

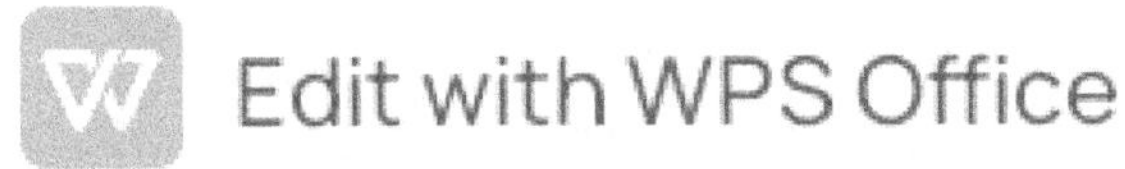

water throughout the day, even if you don't feel thirsty.

3. Check your urine colour

Dark yellow urine suggests dehydration, but pale yellow or clear pee shows enough hydration. Keep an eye on the colour of your urine to quickly determine your hydration levels.

4. Exercise caution with drugs

Some medications might raise the risk of dehydration or disrupt fluid balance in the body. If you are taking any drugs, speak with your doctor about how they may affect your water needs.

5. Consume hydrating foods

Fruits and vegetables high in water content, such as watermelon, cucumbers, oranges, and celery, will help you meet your daily fluid needs. Include these foods in your diet to help you stay hydrated.

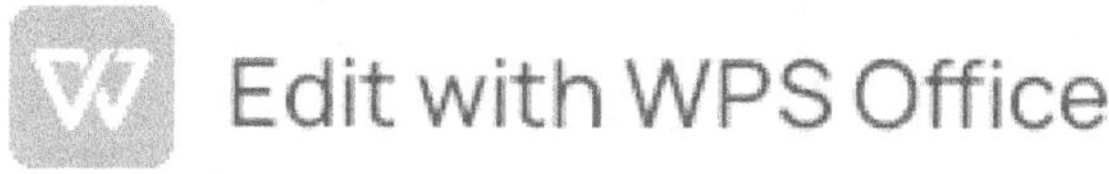

6. Set reminders

If you struggle to remember to drink water throughout the day, try setting reminders on your phone or utilising a water bottle with timers to track your consumption.

Following these hydration principles and prioritising hydration in your daily routine will help you maintain your health, energy levels, and cognitive function as you age. Remember, being hydrated is essential for feeling your best and having a full life. Cheers to excellent health and adequate hydration.

Seniors benefit from paying special attention to nutrients such as potassium, magnesium, and antioxidants. Include potassium-rich foods such as bananas and oranges, magnesium from nuts and seeds, and antioxidants from berries and dark leafy greens. Always seek personalised dietary guidance from a healthcare practitioner.

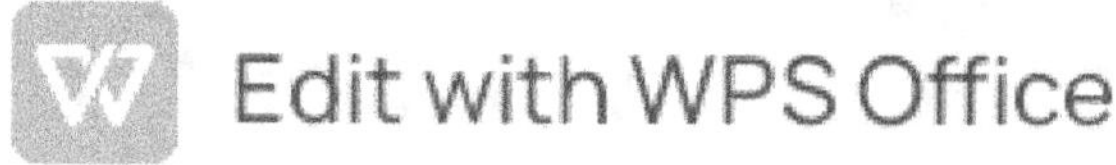

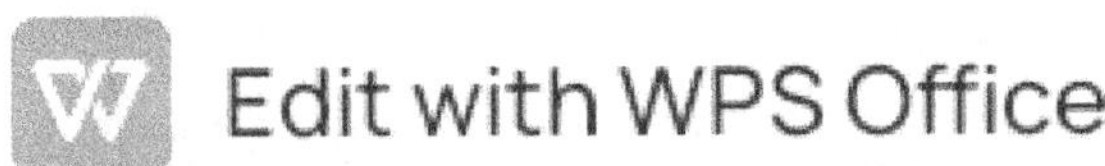

Chapter Eight

Overcoming Challenges and Staying Injury-Free

A. Setting realistic expectations

Setting realistic expectations is critical to achieving success and maintaining a healthy mindset. It's critical to remember that growth takes time and work, and it's acceptable to establish objectives that are difficult yet attainable. Setting reasonable expectations helps you achieve long-term progress while avoiding the traps of disappointment and exhaustion.

When setting expectations for yourself or others, consider the following suggestions:

Be specific

Clarify your aims and objectives to avoid ambiguity and confusion. Specific, quantifiable goals make it easier to monitor progress and alter your plan as necessary.

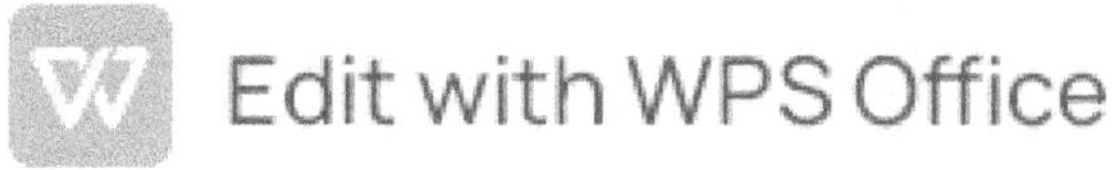

Break it down

Large goals can be overwhelming, so break them down into smaller, more doable activities. This not only makes the objective more attainable, but also gives you a sense of accomplishment along the road.

Consider potential obstacles

Prepare for probable issues and have a plan in place to deal with them. Being prepared for setbacks might help you maintain focus and motivation.

Celebrate Progress

Recognise and celebrate your accomplishments, no matter how minor. Recognising your progress along the way can build your confidence and determination to continue moving forward.

Maintain flexibility

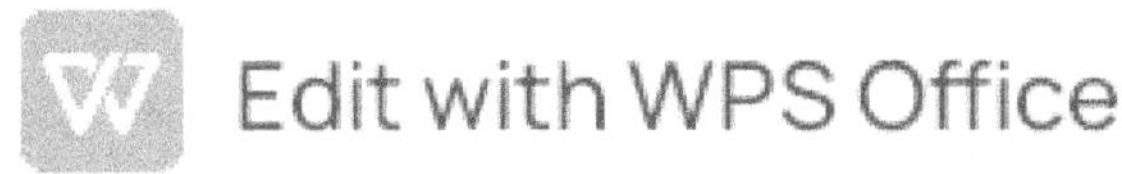

Life is unpredictable, and circumstances can change. Stay adaptive and willing to change your expectations as needed. Remember that it is acceptable to pivot and reassess your goals if necessary.

Setting realistic expectations helps you establish a roadmap for success that is both tough and doable. Remember to be kind to yourself, be patient, and keep going forward one step at a time. You may accomplish great things while retaining a good and healthy mindset if you approach goal setting in a balanced manner. Set realistic goals for yourself and embrace the path ahead to ensure your success.

One of the most difficult problems when beginning an exercise plan is setting unrealistic expectations. It is critical to set attainable goals based on your current fitness level and then progressively grow from there. Setting tiny, realistic benchmarks allows you to track your

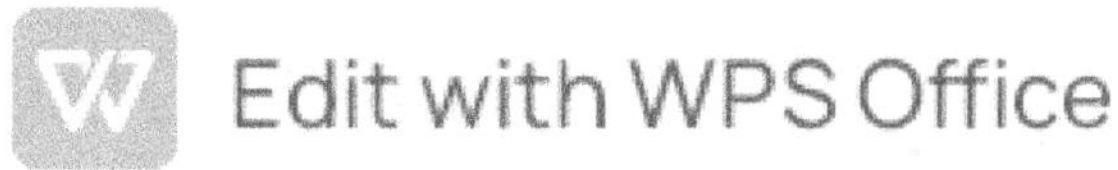

progress and stay encouraged while not placing too much load on your body is Essential

2. Maintaining consistency is essential for avoiding injuries and conquering obstacles. It is critical to start and maintain a consistent fitness schedule. Consistent workouts help your body adapt to the demands placed on it, lowering the risk of injury and enhancing overall performance.

3. Proper Warm-Up and Cool-Down

Many injuries arise as a result of insufficient warm-up or cool-down periods. Before beginning any exercise, you must warm up your muscles and prepare them for the task ahead. This can be accomplished with light cardiovascular workouts, stretching, or even foam rolling. Similarly, cooling down after a workout helps to reduce muscular discomfort and prevent injury.

4. Listen to Your Body

Pay attention to the messages your body sends you when exercising. If you are experiencing pain, discomfort, or weariness that exceeds usual levels, you must listen and respond appropriately. Pushing through pain can result in more severe injuries. To avoid additional injury, practise mindful exercise by noticing any discomfort and changing your practice accordingly.

5. Good Technique and Form

It is worthwhile to devote time and effort to learning the proper posture, alignment, and movement patterns for workouts to maximise benefit while minimising the risk of strains or sprains.

6. Cross-train and Change Your Routine

Overuse injuries are common when doing the same activities repeatedly. To avoid this, incorporate cross-training and change your

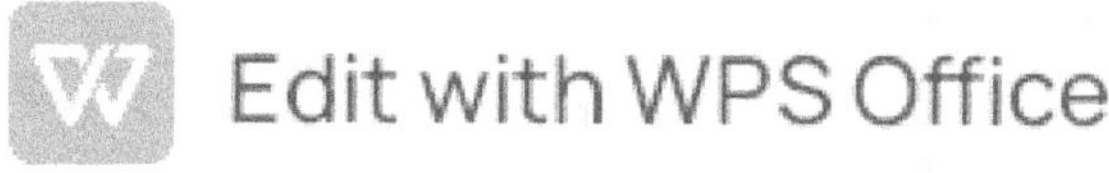

workout routine. Cross-training entails engaging in several forms of physical activity, such as swimming, riding, or yoga, to work different muscle groups and lessen tension in specific sections of the body.

7. Rest and Recovery

Workout Days Your body requires time to heal and rebuild muscular tissue following strenuous activity. Including rest days in your schedule allows your body to recuperate, avoiding overuse problems and maintaining overall fitness levels.

8. Seek Professional Guidance

If you are new to exercising or have special health concerns, you should consult with a trained fitness professional or healthcare provider. They can assist you in developing a customised fitness programme based on your specific demands, ensuring safety, and reducing the chance of injury.

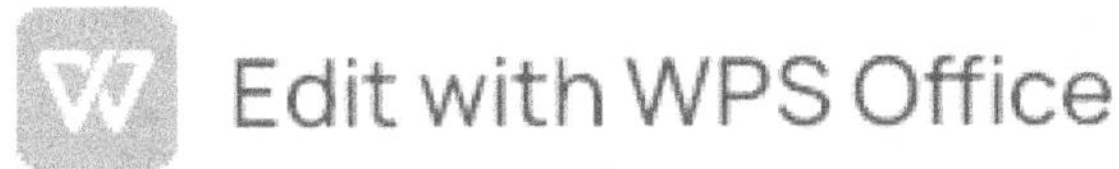

B. Strategies for dealing with time constraints

Break your workouts into shorter periods or add rapid bursts of activity throughout the day.

1. Difficulties with motivation

Set tiny, attainable goals for yourself and reward yourself at each milestone.

2. Modifications for physical limitations

Low-impact alternatives. Swimming and cycling are two hobbies that can help alleviate joint tension.

3. Adaptive equipment

Accept assistive devices or adapted equipment to address physical difficulties.

4. Tailored exercises

Work with a fitness professional to develop personalised programmes that target

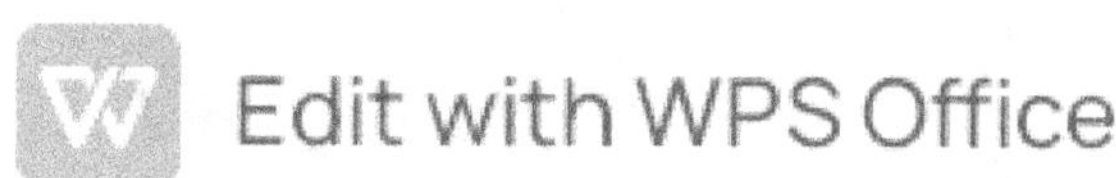

individual constraints.

C. Preventing Injury and Recovery from Setbacks

Warm-up Wisdom.

Make dynamic warm-ups a priority to prepare muscles and joints for activity.

•Smart Progression.

In the vivid tapestry of life, seniors embark on a journey of well-being marked by growth, resilience, and limitless possibility. Smart progression, a beacon of empowerment and vitality, illuminates the route ahead, bringing seniors to optimal health and fulfilment with wisdom and grace.

•Mindful Movement

Smart progression starts with mindful movement, which is a symphony of gentle exercises, stretches, and activities adapted

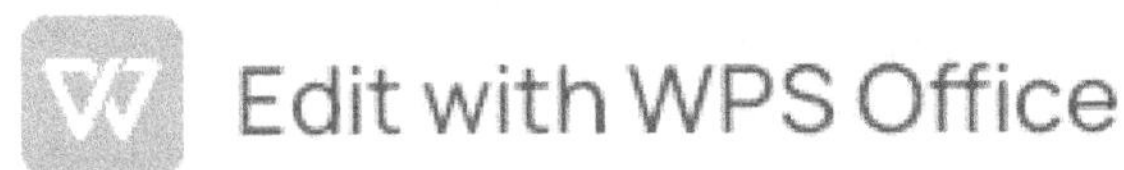

to seniors' specific needs and skills. From yoga and tai chi to walking and swimming, these mindful practices respect the body's rhythms, encouraging flexibility, balance, and energy with each beautiful step.

•**Holistic Health**

Embracing smart progression entails taking a comprehensive approach to health and wellness, nurturing the mind, body, and spirit in harmony. Seniors investigate healthy meals, restorative sleep, and stress-reduction practices to build a strong foundation of well-being and radiate vigour from the inside out.

•**Personalized Pathways**

Smart progression honours the beauty of individuality, recognising each senior's unique path to wellness. Seniors go on a transforming journey of self-discovery, resilience, and empowerment through personalised pathways adapted to their

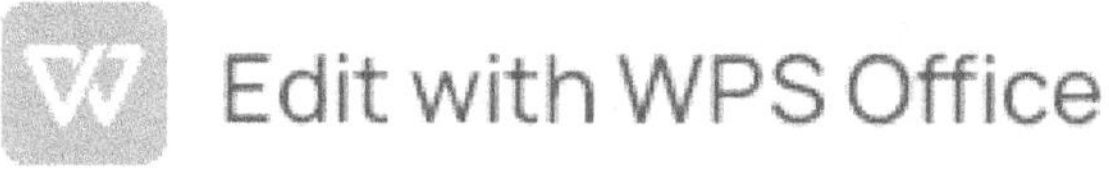

objectives and aspirations, bravely embracing their intrinsic potential.

•Adaptive Advancement

In the ever-changing landscape of well-being, wise progression values adaptive development and the ability to embrace change with resilience. Seniors negotiate life's twists and turns with agility and adaptation, leveraging the power of invention and curiosity to construct new paths to vitality and fulfilment.

•Lifelong Learning

Smart advancement is based on the idea of lifelong learning, which is a spiritual quest for knowledge, growth, and self-discovery. Seniors set out on a path of exploration and discovery, embracing new skills, interests, and passions with infinite curiosity and excitement, enhancing their lives with meaning and delight.

As the tapestry of life unfolds, sensible progression encourages seniors to enjoy the journey with open hearts and minds, celebrating the beauty of each moment and their boundless potential. Seniors go on a revolutionary journey of self-discovery and empowerment, illuminating the route ahead with elegance, resilience, and limitless opportunity.

Rest and Rehabilitation

Allow for enough recuperation time and seek professional help for effective injury rehabilitation. Remember that every step forward represents a win. Adjustments and persistence are essential for overcoming obstacles and cultivating a long-term, injury -free fitness path.

In life, we are continually confronted with trials that test our strength, resilience, and determination. It is at these times of struggle that we have the opportunity to

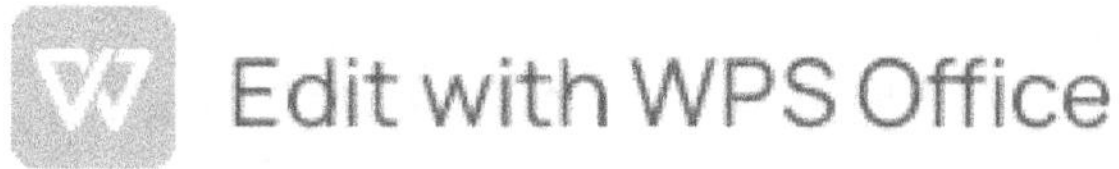

rise above and demonstrate our worth. Whether it's a difficult task at work, a personal difficulty, or a physical impediment, the key to success is our capacity to overcome these challenges with unflinching resolve and a firm focus on our goals.

However, amid the rush and bustle of daily life, it is all too easy to overlook one critical part of self-care: injury prevention. As we push ourselves to new heights and strive for perfection, the possibility of injury looms large, threatening to derail our progress and stymie our accomplishments. But do not worry, there is a method to negotiate this difficult terrain with grace and confidence.

By listening to our body, being aware of our physical limitations, and adding correct stretching, warm-up, and recovery practices into our routines, we may lessen the risk of injury and protect our well-being as we face life's challenges. Let us remember that the

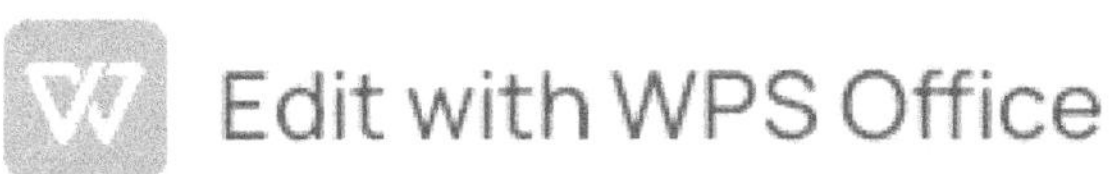

path to success entails not just overcoming obstacles, but also taking care of ourselves along the way.

So, when you go on your path to overcome obstacles and avoid damage, remember this: you are capable, resilient, and have the ability to achieve greatness. Accept the challenges that come your way, overcome them with courage and determination, and always prioritise your health and well-being. With this mindset and approach, there are no limits to what you can do. Keep pushing forward, striving for perfection, and, most importantly, believing in yourself. Your success is waiting for you; go out and claim it!

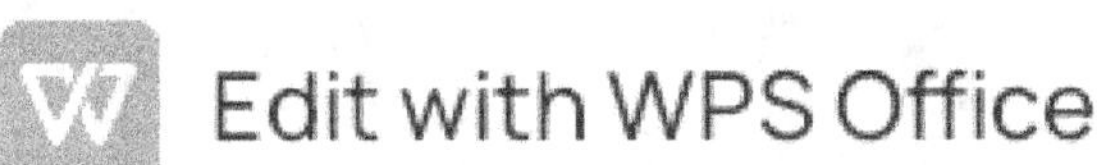

Conclusion: Enhance Your Wellness Symphony.

In conclusion, including exercise in daily life is critical for improving overall health. Following the points given above, individuals can

1.Increase physical strength

Physical strength is more than simply the ability to lift large objects or compete in sports; it is having a healthy and capable physique that can carry us through all areas of our daily life. Increasing physical strength provides numerous physical and mental benefits.

First and foremost, increasing physical strength benefits our general health and well-being. Regular strength training can improve muscle mass, bone density, and joint health. By increasing our strength, we

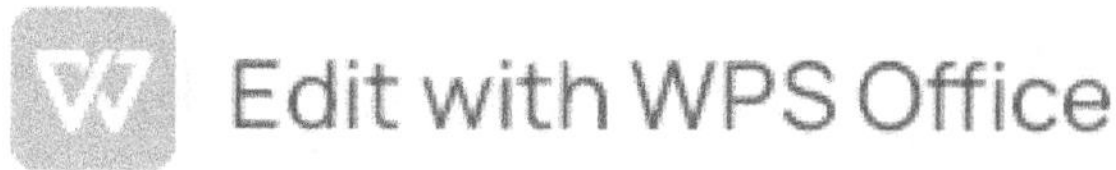

can better support our body's structure and reduce our chances of becoming injured or acquiring certain health disorders like osteoporosis.

Furthermore, physical strength influences our functional capacities. It makes it easier to do ordinary duties like carrying groceries, lifting furniture, and participating in leisure activities. By increasing our physical strength, we can navigate these activities more efficiently and lessen the possibility of straining or harming oneself.

Building physical strength can also help us gain confidence and improve our body image. When we make progress in our strength training journey, we usually feel a sense of success and pride. This positive thinking spreads to other aspects of our lives, increasing self-confidence and self-esteem.

Increasing physical strength also has

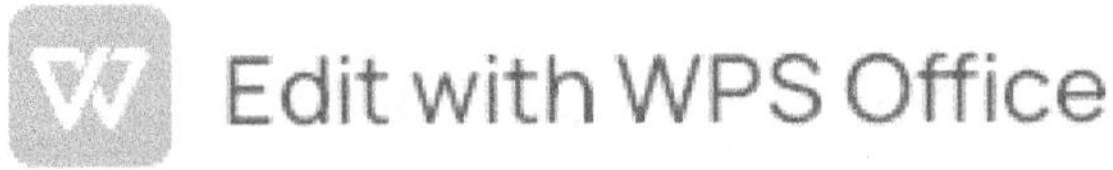

positive effects on mental health. Exercise, including weight training, has been shown to increase endorphin levels, which are natural mood boosters. Regular physical activity can help to alleviate stress, anxiety, and depressive symptoms. A healthy mind and a strong physical body work together to improve one's overall quality of life.

To begin building physical strength, participate in activities that stress your muscles and gradually raise your training intensity over time. Incorporate workouts like weightlifting, resistance training, and bodyweight movements into your fitness regimen. To avoid overexertion or injury, listen to your body and allow yourself rest and recuperation time.

To summarise, improving physical strength is a worthwhile investment in our general well-being. It not only improves our physical health and functional capacities, but also has a great impact on our mental health

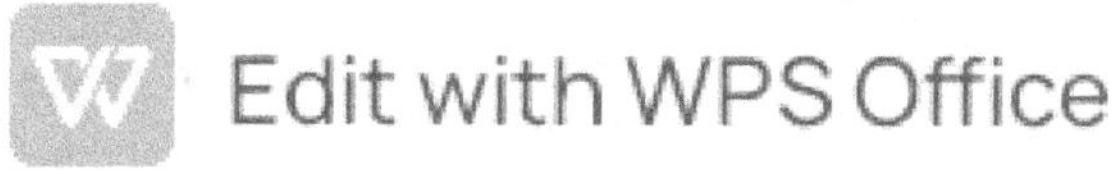

and confidence. As a result, let us prioritise strength training and reap the numerous benefits it provides to our life.

2. Improve general health

Taking care of our health is critical to our general well-being and happiness. By consciously working to improve our overall health, we can improve our physical, mental, and emotional well-being, resulting in a higher quality of life.

Maintaining a balanced and nutritious diet is an important step towards improving overall health. Eating a variety of fruits, vegetables, whole grains, lean proteins, and healthy fats gives our bodies the nutrition they need to function properly. Furthermore, staying hydrated is critical for normal body functions and general wellness. We may strengthen our immune system, increase our energy levels, and lower our chance of developing chronic diseases by eating

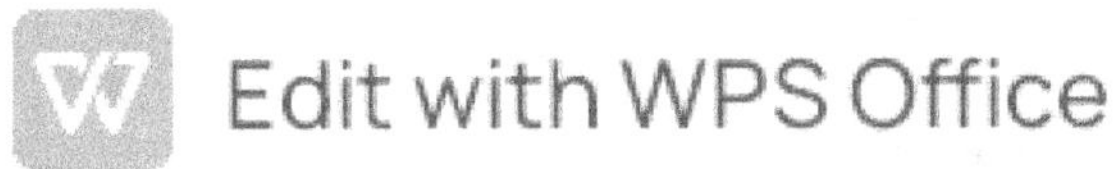

healthy and staying hydrated.

Regular physical activity is another important aspect of boosting overall health. Exercising not only helps to maintain our bodies in shape, but it also provides several health benefits. Physical activity helps with weight management, muscle and bone strength, cardiovascular health, and mental clarity and mood. Simply introducing moderate-intensity exercises into our everyday routines, such as walking, running, cycling, or dancing, can significantly improve our health.

Furthermore, stress management is essential for boosting overall health. Chronic stress can harm our physical and mental well-being, resulting in a variety of health problems. Finding good coping skills, such as mindfulness, relaxation techniques, or hobbies, can help us minimise stress and maintain a sense of calm and balance in our life. It is critical to prioritise self-care

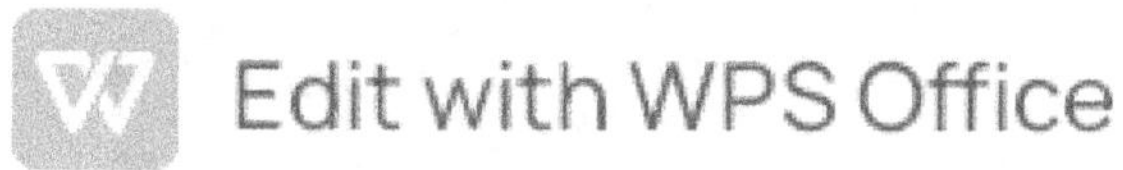

and allocate time for activities that bring us joy and relaxation.

In addition, obtaining enough sleep is an important part of improving overall health. Sleep allows our bodies and minds to relax, mend, and renew. Aim for seven to nine hours of quality sleep per night to maintain peak physical and cognitive function. Establishing a consistent sleep schedule and providing a soothing sleep environment might help improve sleep habits.

Finally, regular check-ups and screenings with healthcare specialists are essential for preserving and monitoring our health. These preventive methods aid in detecting potential health issues early on, allowing for timely intervention and treatment. To stay in good health, we must prioritise frequent medical and dental checkups.

To summarise, promoting overall health is a multidimensional endeavour that affects

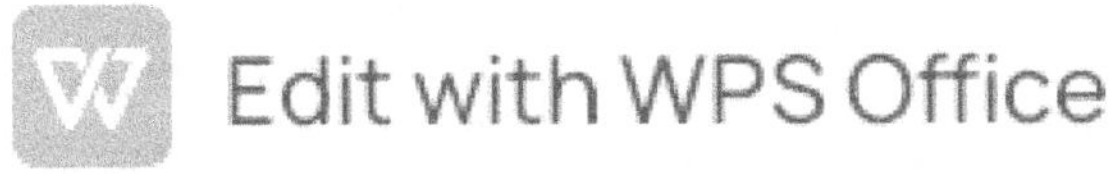

many facets of our lives. We may improve our general health by eating well, exercising regularly, controlling stress, getting enough sleep, and seeking regular medical treatment. Let us put our health first and make intentional decisions that lead to a healthier and happier life.

3. Increase confidence

Regular exercise not only improves physical appearance, but it also increases self-esteem and confidence.

Age is not a barrier to confidence; rather, it reflects a life full of experience, wisdom, and endurance. As seniors, your path is rich with stories, each adding depth and character to your unique tapestry.

Embracing confidence is acknowledging the invaluable wealth of information and insight you possess. It's about honouring your accomplishments, big and little, and acknowledging the inner strength you

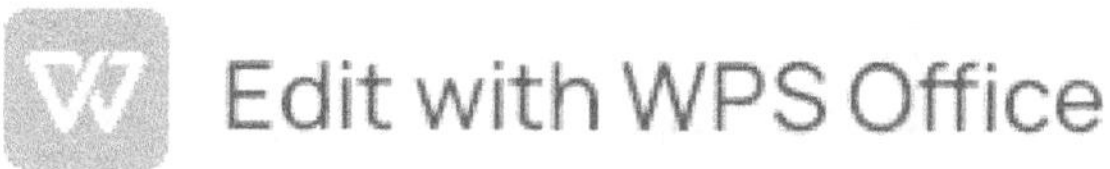

possess.

With each laugh line and beautiful step, you emanate a dazzling confidence that illuminates the world around you. Your presence reflects a life well lived, full of joy, victory, and development.

So stand tall, accept your wisdom, and let your confidence shine through. Your path is inspiring, and your spirit is unlimited. With each new day, may you walk with grace, courage, and a firm trust in the beauty of your existence.

4. Find enjoyable activities

In the rush and bustle of daily life, it's easy to become engrossed in commitments and responsibilities, overlooking the simple pleasure of participating in fun activities. However, finding joy in what we do is critical to our general well-being and

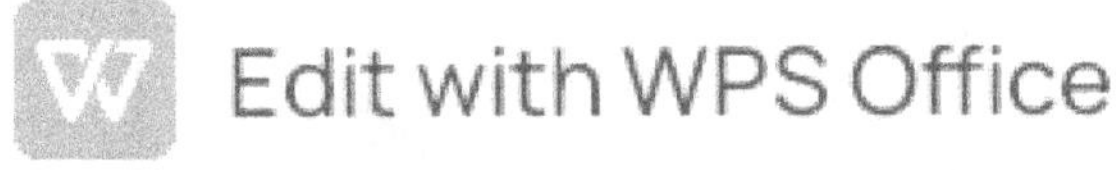

happiness.

Seeking for interesting things does not have to be hard or expensive. It might be as simple as rediscovering old hobbies, pursuing new interests, or spending time outdoors. The trick is to focus on activities that bring us actual enjoyment and fulfilment.

Engaging in interesting activities provides numerous rewards. It is a sort of self-care that allows us to refresh and renew our brains and bodies. It can also serve as a great stress reliever, providing moments of reprieve from the stresses of everyday life.

Furthermore, pleasant hobbies have the ability to improve creativity, happiness, and general quality of life. These moments of joy, whether they be cooking a favourite meal, learning a musical instrument, or going on a leisurely walk, enrich and provide purpose to our lives.

Incorporating fun things into our daily routine is a purposeful decision that takes planning and effort. It entails putting our personal pleasure first and making time for the activities that bring us joy, even in the middle of hectic schedules and competing expectations.

As we manage life's difficulties, let us not lose sight of the value of finding joy in the simplest moments. Let us make time for delightful activities, savouring each moment and cultivating our sense of well-being. As a result, we cultivate a life rich in moments of happiness, contentment, and fulfilment.

5. Make tiny changes to daily habits.

Adding exercise to your daily routine can be as simple as taking the stairs instead of the lift or walking instead of driving short distances.

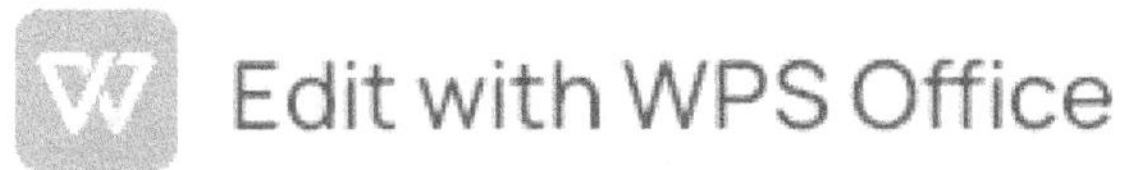

6. Seek support

As seniors face the myriad challenges and transitions that come with ageing, seeking help becomes a vital resource in their quest for health, happiness, and fulfilment. From physical health difficulties to mental well-being, seniors can benefit greatly from accessing support networks suited to their requirements.

Healthcare Professionals

Building solid relationships with healthcare professionals is critical for elders' general well-being. Regular check-ups, preventive screenings, and open communication with doctors and specialists can assist in addressing medical issues, managing chronic illnesses, and promoting good ageing.

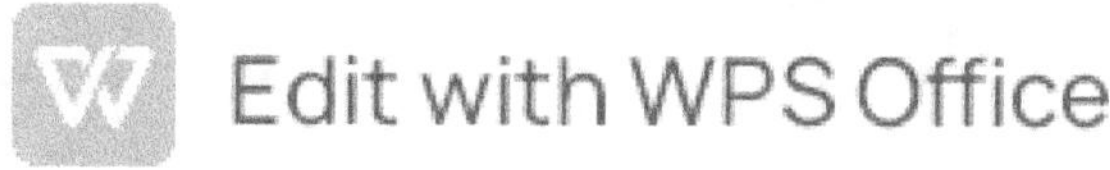

Community Resources

Community organisations, senior centres, and local support groups provide a multitude of resources and services tailored to seniors' various needs. These community resources promote connection, involvement, and a sense of belonging by providing meal assistance and transportation services, as well as social activities and educational sessions.

Family & Friends

Support from family members, friends, and carers is critical to seniors' emotional and social well-being. Building strong ties and having open lines of communication with loved ones can give seniors a solid support network to rely on in times of need and celebration.

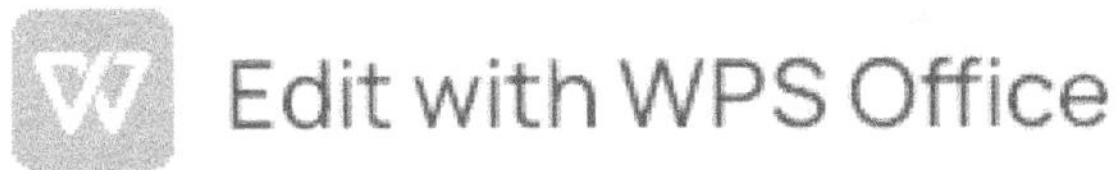

Mental Health Professional

Addressing mental health difficulties is also critical for seniors' overall quality of life. Accessing mental health services, such as counselling, therapy, and support groups, can assist seniors in coping with stress, anxiety, sadness, grief, and other emotional issues, fostering resilience and emotional well-being.

Technology and TeleHealth

Technology has changed the way elders receive support services by providing virtual platforms for telehealth appointments, online support groups, and remote counselling sessions. Embracing technology enables seniors to communicate with experts and peers, access essential resources, and receive assistance from the comfort and safety of their own homes.

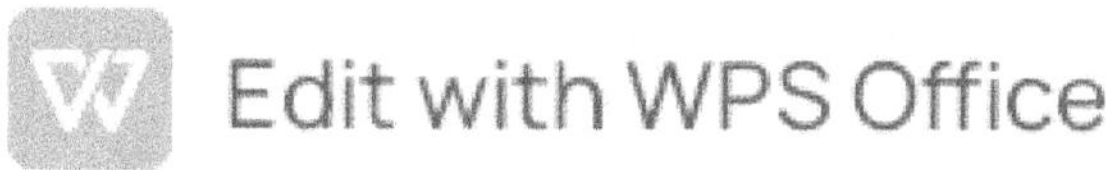

Encouraging seniors to seek help enables them to proactively address their needs, confidently handle life transitions, and preserve a sense of independence and autonomy as they age. We develop a culture of compassion, empathy, and inclusivity, resulting in a supportive environment in which elders can thrive, prosper, and live their best lives.

7. Use technology

Incorporating technology into seniors' exercise routines can change the way they engage in physical activity, benefiting their health, independence, and general well-being. With technological improvements, seniors now have access to a diverse set of tools and services to help and enhance their fitness journey.

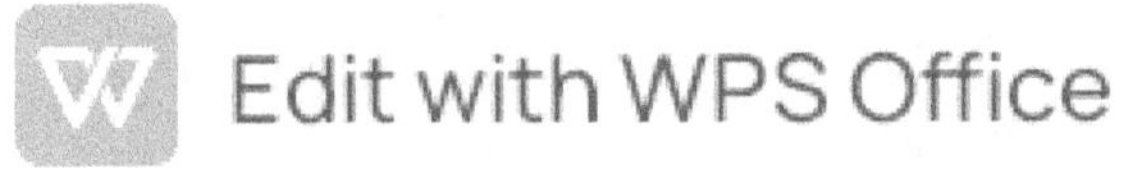

Fitness Apps and Wearable Devices

Fitness applications and wearable gadgets provide seniors with customised workout plans, step tracking, heart rate monitoring, and even mild reminders to be active throughout the day. These tools provide useful insights into their progress, allowing users to create attainable goals and track their progress over time.

Virtual Exercise Classes

Virtual exercise sessions bring the gym experience straight to seniors' homes, providing a range of workout options based on their fitness level and interests. From yoga and tai chi to strength training and aerobics, seniors can pick from a variety of sessions offered by licensed teachers, all from the comfort and safety of their own homes.

Gamification in Exercise

Gamification gives a sense of pleasure and excitement to seniors' fitness routines, encouraging them to stay active and engaged. Health games and challenges promote friendly competition, social contact, and a sense of accomplishment as seniors strive to meet their health goals.

Remote monitoring and telehealth

Remote monitoring gadgets and telehealth services allow elders to receive personalised feedback and coaching from healthcare specialists, ensuring that they exercise safely and successfully. Seniors may stay connected with their healthcare team and make educated exercise decisions thanks to virtual consultations and remote vital sign monitoring.

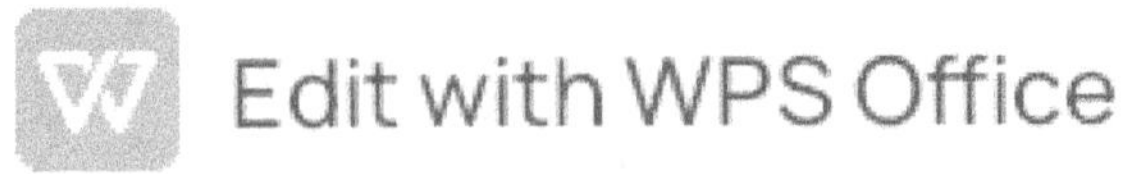

Social Connectivity

Technology promotes social connectivity among seniors by allowing them to interact with classmates, friends, and family members who have similar health goals and interests. Online forums, social networking platforms, and video conferencing tools help seniors stay connected, motivated, and accountable as they begin their exercise journey.

By embracing technology, seniors can overcome exercise hurdles, stay motivated, and feel more empowered and independent in managing their health and well-being. With the correct tools and assistance, technology may alter seniors' exercise experiences, allowing them to live happier, healthier, and more satisfying lives.

8.Recognise and accept your body's limitations

In a world that often emphasises pushing

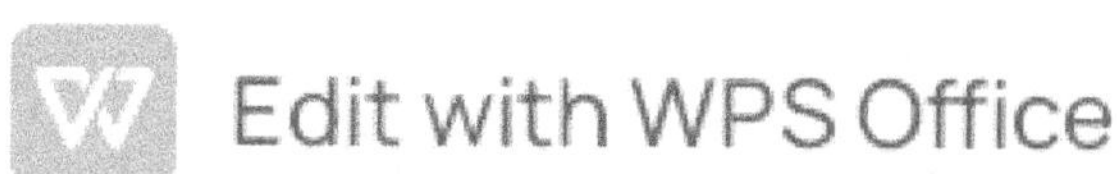

boundaries and exceeding limits, acknowledging and respecting our bodies' limitations is extremely valuable. Our bodies are magnificent vessels, each uniquely built with its own set of capabilities and limitations. However, in our quest of productivity, success, and societal standards, we frequently ignore or discard these fundamental constraints.

Recognising our bodies' limitations is not a sign of weakness; rather, it demonstrates knowledge and self-awareness. It is about knowing and honouring our physical form's inherent restrictions. Our bodies, like machines, can only operate within specific limitations without incurring damage. Beyond those limits, they may falter or become vulnerable.

Recognising our body's limitations helps us understand what activities and lifestyles are sustainable and nutritious for us. It enables us to make informed choices about how we

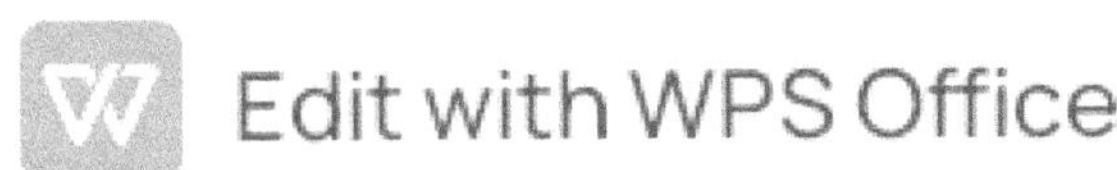

spend our time, energy, and resources. Whether it's recognising the need for proper relaxation after periods of effort or grasping the necessity of pacing ourselves during physical activities, this awareness enables us to prioritise our health.

Acceptance is an important aspect of this process. It is about accepting our bodies precisely as they are, with all of their strengths and limitations. Acceptance does not imply resignation or complacency; rather, it is a state of self-compassion and self-care. It entails letting go of unreasonable expectations and cultural pressures in favour of growing a genuine respect for our bodies and everything they enable us to experience.

Furthermore, understanding our body's limitations promotes resilience and adaptation. It encourages us to work with our bodies rather than against them, finding innovative methods to overcome obstacles

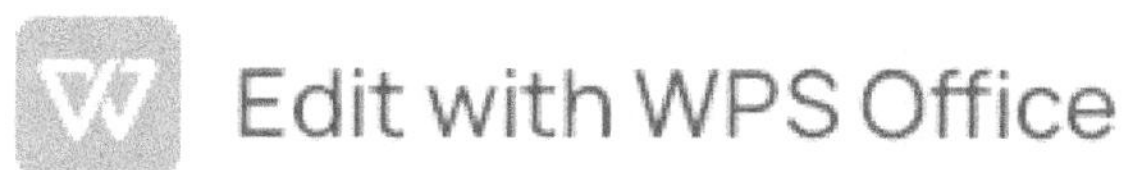

and achieve our goals in ways that respect our well-being. It also allows us to consider other paths and techniques that may be more in line with our physical abilities and goals.

In a world that frequently promotes pushing through pain and dismissing signs of anguish, accepting our body's limitations is a radical act of self-love. It's about listening to our bodies' whispers before they become yells, and responding with respect and compassion. It is about understanding that our worth is established not by our productivity or ability to achieve artificial criteria, but by our potential for self-awareness, compassion, and growth.

 Modifying workouts or getting professional assistance as needed guarantees safety and avoids injuries.

 Individuals who follow these ideas can develop a long-term fitness regimen that

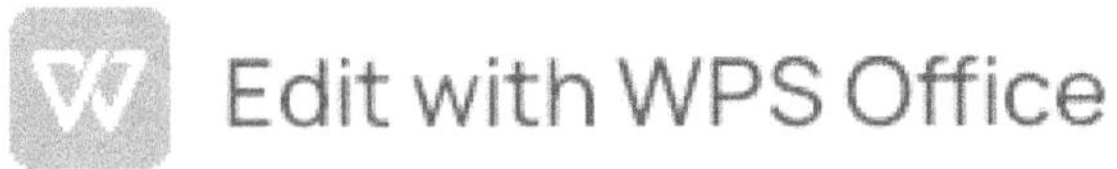

becomes an intrinsic part of their daily lives, resulting in enhanced physical and mental health. Accept the route to good health and make fitness a lifelong commitment.

Remember that wellbeing is not a destination, but rather a harmonic rhythm of choices.

From overcoming time constraints to creating specialised exercises and persevering in the face of disappointments, your fitness journey is a celebration of tiny and large accomplishments.

Savour the thrill of every step as you lace on your trainers and celebrate your sweat-soaked victories. Whether you are overcoming obstacles, adjusting movements, or advocating for injury prevention, you are all part of your personal health symphony.

To summarise, acknowledging and accepting our body's limitations is a

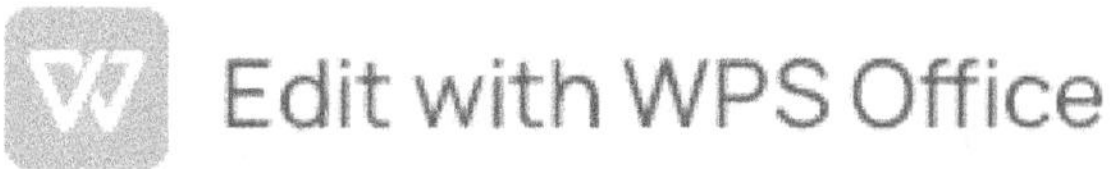

significant act of self-discovery and empowerment. It encourages us to develop a greater connection with ourselves, to respect our bodies' knowledge, and to live in accordance with our deepest wants and goals. By doing so, we provide the groundwork for a life that is not just sustainable and fulfilling, but also deeply nourishing and delightful.

So turn up the heat, embrace the obstacles with a smile, and let your fitness mojo shine. Your wellness journey is a constantly developing masterpiece, with you as the maestro orchestrating vitality, power, and confidence. Let the beat continue, and may your wellness melody be filled with the colourful echoes of a healthier, happier you.